Let's
EAT
Mindfully

*UPDATED

Jim Painter, PhD RD

with Rosemary Painter, MSEd

Special Thanks

To Rosemary, my wife, companion, support co-writer and editor who was always there to encourage me to keep writing. To Xinyue Wang my student assistant who created numerous graphs and charts and found information buried in governmental documents. To Maggie Schuster who also aided in documenting and referencing. To all my students over the years that conducted the many of the studies reported in this book. Thank you all. And most importantly to our great God Who is the reason for life itself.

Let's
EAT
Mindfully

*UPDATED

by Jim Painter, PhD, RD

with Rosemary Painter, MSEd

ISBN 13: 978-172-8823393

          www.drjimpainter.com

Table of Contents

Section I: The Problem

Obesity has been increasing worldwide for the past several decades and is still going up. During the 25 years from the mid-1970s to 2000, obesity doubled in the US for adults age 18-64. Yet for hundreds of years before the last quarter of the 20th century obesity was not a major issue.

Obesity by age, US, 1971-1974 through 2005-2006

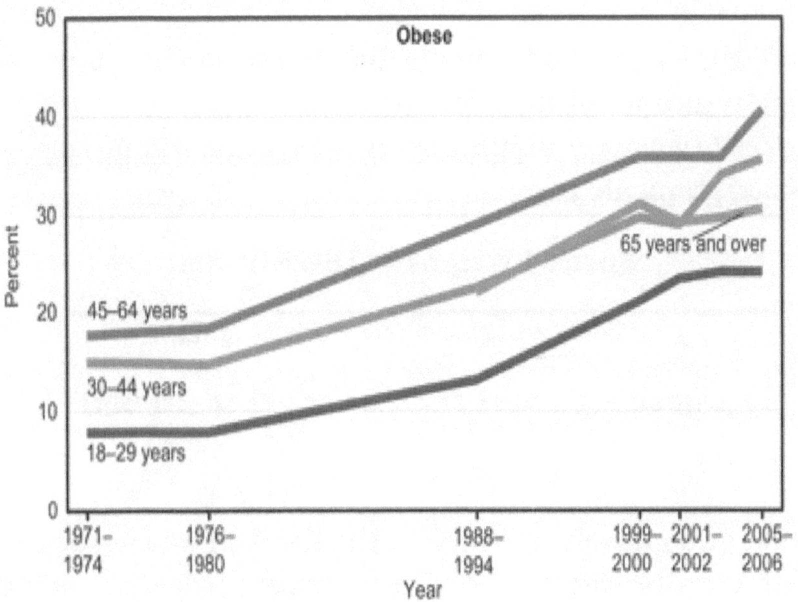

NCHS, Obesity – Americans still growing, but not as fast. (n.d.). Retrieved

Let's start with a definition of obesity. We have standard weight charts for healthy living. A healthy normal adult weight is between 18.5 – 24.9 body mass index (BMI). This calculation can be done by your physician, but it is a simple mathematical formula to calculate your own BMI:

body weight in kilograms ÷ (height in meters)^2

Or even easier, go to this website and type in your height and weight.
https://www.nhlbi.nih.gov/health/educational/lose_wt/BMI/bmicalc.htm

Normal weight = 18-24.9 BMI.

Overweight = 25 – 29.9 BMI.

Obese = greater than or equal to 30 BMI.

Most of us have some idea of the health risks associated with obesity and yet those don't necessarily dissuade us from overeating. Despite the risks of heart disease, cancer, sleep apnea, type 2 diabetes, stroke and more, in the moment of consumption, those concerns seem far away and much less important than treating ourselves, being hospitable, easily convinced or simply mindless about what we eat.

As with adults, obesity rates are increasing among youth in the US: 13% in 1999 and 17% in 2013. During the same 25-year period from the mid-1970s to 2000, obesity more than doubled for children and adolescents. And there are suggestions that obesity in childhood can lead to a shortened lifespan along with many other health problems.

But there is a bright spot in the obesity epidemic: the Women, Infants and Children program (WIC). WIC works with children 2-4 years old and WIC data in 2008 showed that 15 states had obesity rates greater than 16% but by 2010 it was only 14 states and by 2012, only 10 states had 16% of children categorized as obese. Hats off to the WIC program!

Trends of Obesity in the U.S. WIC children 2-4 years

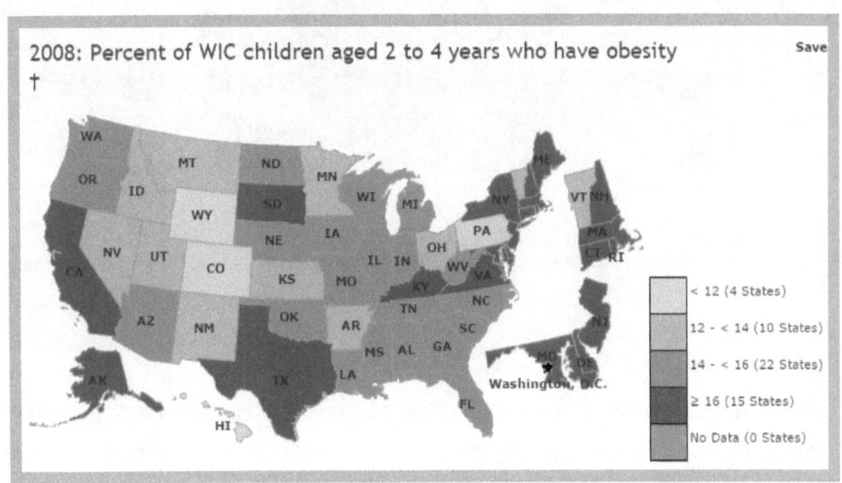

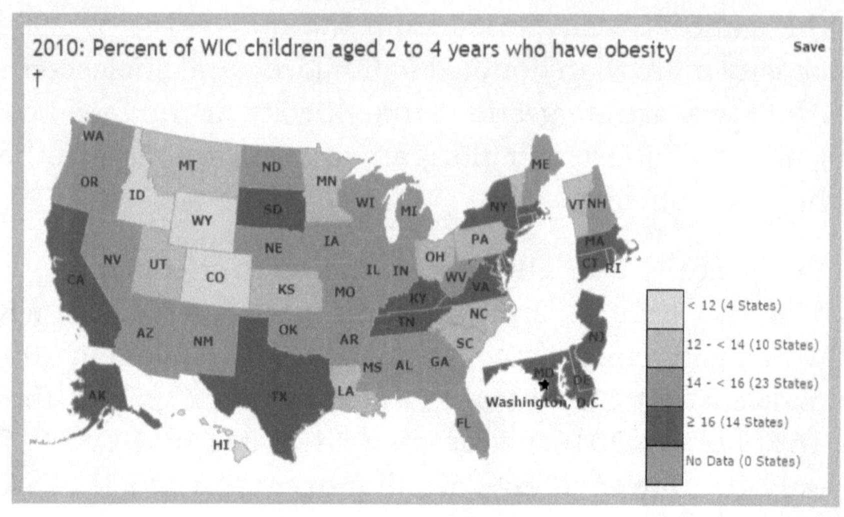

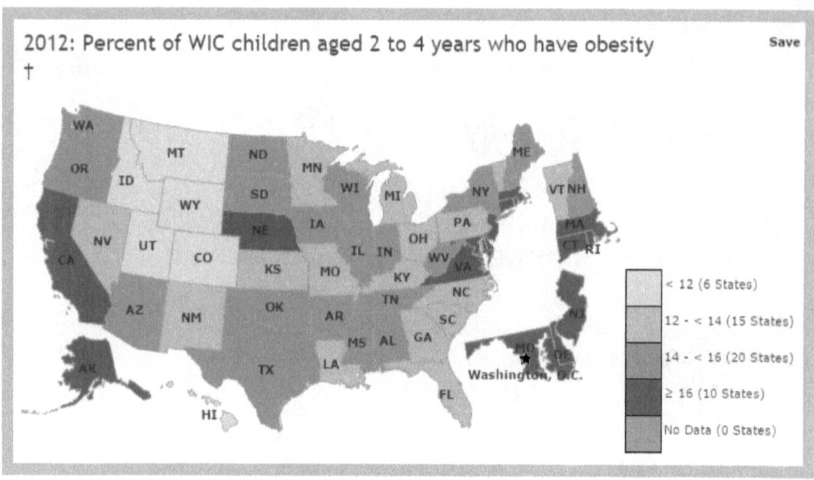

Although the US boasts one of the highest obesity rates, obesity is a worldwide problem. In this chart below from the World Health Organization we can see the darker shading represents over 30% of the population as obese.

Worldwide Prevalence of Obesity, Ages 18+

2010-2014

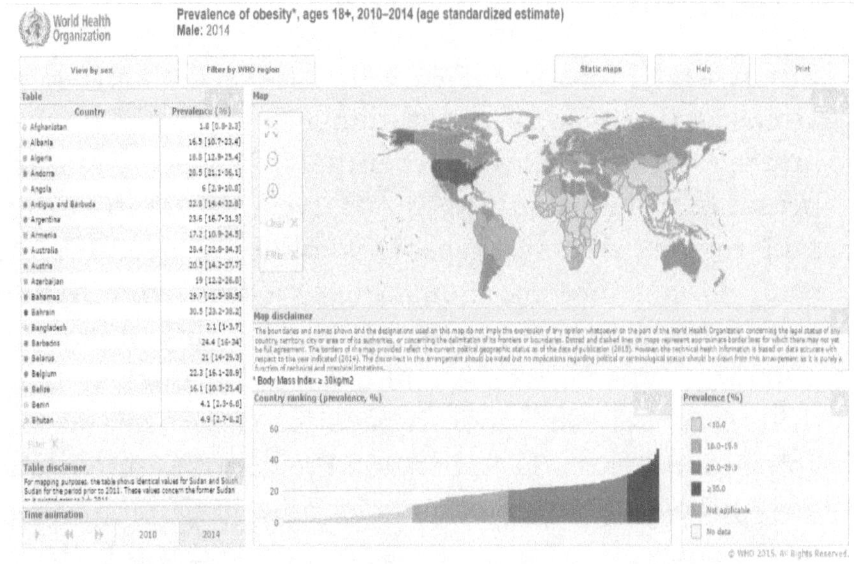

World Health Organization

Before the mid-1970s Americans typically were a normal weight. What has caused the recent increase in obesity? When I ask people during my lectures, they often give me the same answers: lack of exercise, sedentary lifestyles, stress and pressure, advertising, genetics or deep emotional needs. These are certainly associated with obesity, but my question is: which of these have changed in the past four decades and are associated with the rapid increase in obesity?

Lifestyle and lack of exercise? True enough, we have

more technology that lends us to ease and yet, we were couch potatoes in the 1970's. If we look at lifestyles in the last few decades, they haven't changed so much as to cause this doubling of obesity.

Stress and Pressure? We were stressed then; we are stressed now. Every generation faces certain stresses and pressures; these are perennials. We face stress and pressure from situations in our lives, things in our city and region, stresses regarding national agendas and even global concerns. Sometimes we think that NOW is worse than any other time, but in all reality, it is not so different. When I was a child, we did a nuclear bomb drill in school every month because the Russians were going to nuke us. Then in 1962 President Kennedy shot a round over the bow of a Soviet ship in Cuba and said to the effect, "One more advance and you will be blown out of the water." That was pretty stressful and could have started World War III. Although the more recent terrorism is indeed stressful, our obesity trends cannot be laid at the feet of this ancient yet modern day threat.

Does advertising compel people to buy? Indeed, it can! Even if it is a subliminal message, we might opt to buy a food that sounds good in that moment. However, was there not advertising in the 1970's? Yes, and plenty of it. We cannot lay the whole of obesity on the fact of clever marketing and advertising. Yet, we do need to be mindful of what messages we hear and see, and what we permit to influence our lives.

Genetics: Do they play a part? Yes, genetics definitely play a part in who might be predisposed to overweight or even obesity, but it is not a guarantor of that outcome. Further, the genetics handed down from generation to generation haven't changed enough to cause this hyper- and relatively sudden rise in obesity. When we look at TV programs and movies from 30-50 years ago, most of the actors and actresses are amazingly thin by today's standards. Dick Van Dyke, and Michael Landon look skinny. Even the tough guys in that era like Steve McQueen, Charlton Heston, Clint Eastwood and Sean Connery as 007 look thin by today's standards. On the program, Bonanza, we used to think Hoss was a huge character, but in seeing a re-run of that program, he looks normal and the others look very slight. We have become accustomed to larger people to the extent that we now fail to recognize a healthy weight when we see it! Genetics impact all aspects of health, but they haven't changed to that extent in the past 40 years to cause obesity to rise to over one third of our population.

Finally, we all know some emotional eaters and likely have personally had moments of emotional eating. This usually goes back to perceived stress or pressure which was addressed before. Were there only a few emotional eaters in the 90's but now more than 1 in 3 people feel so emotionally overwhelmed as to cause obesity? If we answer yes, we have far more problems than this book can address.

The premise of this book is that the current obesity epidemic has been undergirded and preceded by two recent phenomena; food is everywhere and portions are bigger, plus we lose track of how much we eat. We lose track inadvertently by mindlessly munching, encouraged by availability, suggestion and environment. As we become more mindful of food options and recognize our choices, we can opt into a healthy calorie intake and a healthier life.

Section II: The Genesis of the Problem

Food is Everywhere

It didn't use to be so. We used to be able to drive down the street and not be confronted with thousands of eating possibilities within a few hundred yards. We used to drive into a gas station and the options were to buy gasoline, oil for the car and cigarettes. Now, the convenience store has replaced the repair shop and with that convenience comes endless opportunity for mindless consumption. Most of the foods you walk past in order to pay for gas are high-calorie, low-nutrient dense foods.

Further, we can pull into fast food outlets conveniently located and without even the effort of exiting the car, can order 1,500-2,000 calories worth of food and then eat it in just a few minutes. That was not the case 40-50 years ago. There were "blue laws" or social norms which prevented most establishments from being open on Sundays, including most restaurants. In the age when women went from homemakers to bringing home a paycheck, fewer and fewer wanted to come home from a hard day's work and then prepare a meal for the family. Restaurants have multiplied to serve the ever busy, don't-wish-to-cook crowd and the social taboos of not cooking for oneself went by the wayside.

So within this environment of abundance, where food is everywhere and portions are bigger, quickly purchased and quickly consumed, what are we to do?

For some of us, overeating has become a way of life. Although food is everywhere, if we are aware of the relatively recent changes in the food environment, there are techniques we can use to help us eat less even in this abundance.

Portions are Bigger

People sit down at a meal and exclaim, "This is enough for two people!" and then proceed to try to finish it all singlehandedly. Why do restaurants give us so much? One reason is that the cost of preparing larger portions is very small and it increases consumer's feeling of value and satisfaction. We are generally wowed by receiving plenty, but if our portion is appropriate or even small, we tend to think negatively of it. We seem to want to have feast days far too frequently! Portions served and sold have increased over the past two decades. A Hershey chocolate bar was originally 0.6 oz. and now they can be up to half a pound. We have all seen those giant half- pound bars in stores and buy them because we are cheap and thrifty. We get more candy for the dollar and imagine that this half pound candy bar is going to last us for a week. But what tends to happen is we sit down in front of the TV and take a bite or break off a few squares. That was a great bite! Then we think, "I'm going to have just one more bite." Within 30 minutes, the program is over and we have consumed a half a pound of chocolate. It was not our goal and we didn't intend to, but we ate it all mindlessly. We were fooled by not recognizing what proper portions are.

This distortion of portions can be found in so many examples: beer, burgers, grandma's cooking, eating out... it's the same. While our thirst could be quenched with 8 or 12 oz., we opt for the large – and to make it worse, many venues don't even offer an option as small as 12 ounces anymore.

Food/ Beverage	Intro- duction	Size at intro (ounces)	2002 sizes (ounces)
Budweiser	**1936**	7.0	**7, 12, 22, 40**
Hershey bar	**1908**	0.6	**1.6, 2.6, 4.0, 7.0, 8.0**
BK fry	**1954**	2.6	**2.6, 4.1, 5.7, 6.9**
McD burger	**1955**	1.6	**1.6, 3.2, 4.0, 8.0**
Soda-BK	**1954**	12.0, 16.0	**12.0, 16.0, 22.0, 32.0, 42.0**

Young & Nestle, 2003. JADA Expanding Portion Sizes in the US Marketplace. (231-234)

Here are a few examples of how our portions have changed over time.

A cookie from 20 years ago was 50 calories. Today's cookies can easily be several hundred calories. Same with cheesecake which was 260 calories per serving and is now 500-600 calories. Muffins used to be fairly small – about 1.5 oz. and 200 calories, and now they are frequently 4 oz. and easily 500 calories.

Similarly, bagels have also gotten bigger. They used to be about 140 calories and now they are about 350 calories. I know so many people who feel pleased with themselves for having a bagel for breakfast (perhaps because a bagel is not sugar coated like a donut and is fat free.) "All I had today for breakfast was a bagel." But do these people eat the bagel dry? No, we all tend to put fatty cream cheese or sweet jam on them. And we are often lavish with ourselves. Not just a tad of jam or cream cheese, but we slathered it on! Do they realize that this 350-calorie bagel now may be soaring to 500-800 calories and the same carbohydrate content as 3 - 4 slices of bread?

We are fooled by portion! We think we are eating a simple little bagel for breakfast, but we can consume nearly half of the calories needed all day.

Burgers are the same way. Burgers from 20 years ago were about 300 calories. Now the average burger is approximately 600 calories and there are some on the market at nearly 1,500 calories. The Monster Burger has 1,420 calories! That is just the burger, not including the calories from the fries and drink that come with it! Do people usually ask for a small fry with that? No, they want value for their money. But small fries have about 200 calories; large fries may be 600 calories. Now that 1,400 calorie meals is about 2000 calories! And if you have a milk shake with that, it adds another 1,000 calories or so to the already huge total. The single meal can be in the neighborhood of 3,000 calories!

Here's the problem with food -- it always digests! Within four to six hours, your body or society will tell you it's time to eat again! We remember that at lunch we had a huge burger/fries/shake so we decide not to have dessert with dinner. We would need to skip dinner, breakfast and then skip dessert at lunch the next day to offset that huge calorie intake of the previous lunch!

Value Marketing

There was a documentary put out some years ago called *Super Size Me*. What the program intended to do was to end fast food, but what it did was kill the use of the word *Super Size* in the menu marketing of fast foods. Instead, the industry started using words such as *Value Sized* or *Combo Meal*. Value marketing would connote getting a lot more product for a relatively small raise in price. Companies do this because they make more money at it, not because you need more food!   The question we need to be asking is: Is it of value to us personally to get more of something that we didn't need in the first place?

My example: I want to hang a picture on the wall, so I go to the store to purchase a small hammer for the job.

When I get to the check-out with my little hammer, the cashier says, "I have a deal for you! For just 25¢ more, you can purchase this big sledge hammer." But I don't really need a sledge hammer, just the small one will do. The cashier pressed the issue and the banner overhead screamed "Value."   We get enthralled with the big hammer and get it, take it home, smash a hole in the wall, lose the nail in the wall, bloody our thumb, all because the sledgehammer was too big for the job!   But it had value at the moment of purchase!   So value marketing is something we need to be mindful of as we are purchasing food.

One day, I was at a Chick-fil-A buying a sandwiches for the extended family, when the cashier said to me, "Would you like to make the sandwiches combo meals." Following my own theory, I said, "No" but then the cashier blindsided me with, "It's free." What? For no extra price, I get lattice fries and a drink? I asked how that was possible and she told me it was part of a promotion. Finally getting tired of my shock, she said again, "Do you want it or not?"   I hung my head and said, "Okay." How can I say "No" to free food?! So when I returned to the family, my daughter-in-law saw me with all the fries and drinks and said, "What happened to Dad?!"

I fell for it because it was free! It wasn't even a little extra! And yet, none of us needed the extra calories of the fries and drinks.   So we must be mindful of value marketing ahead of time so that we can have the possibility of resisting it. Remembering our value - what is valuable to us - in that moment rather than being compelled to go against our better choice is key:

Mindfulness!

What do you get with value marketing? Typically, by getting the side and the drink that accompanies an item in a combo or value, you will add an extra 600 calories to the meal. Remember, what value is it to get something that you didn't need in the first place? When was the last time you said, "Wow, the day has gone badly; if I could just find an extra 600 calories for cheap (or free) that would help me!"

If you ingested an extra 600 calories a day and never compensated for it by cutting back to that same degree later that day or the next day, that would add up to about a pound per week. In a year, that would be over 50 pounds!

It's not just fast food, but regular restaurants do the same thing. A plate of spaghetti served at a restaurant 30 years ago was about 500 calories; now it is usually over 1,000. What can we do to help ourselves to be mindful when we eat?

It's not just restaurants, but even the food we buy at the grocery store or convenience store comes in ever-increasing portions. At 7-11 you can get a Gulp size drink at 20 oz. and 200 calories, the Big Gulp at 30 oz. and 300 calories, the Super Gulp at 40 oz. and 400 calories and the Double Gulp is 50 oz. and over 500 calories and now they have the Extreme Gulp which has simply way too many calories.

Even the Tollhouse cookie recipe, though it hasn't changed in sixty years, now serves 60, whereas, when it was created, it made 100 cookies. Why is that? ...To save your relationships, of course! People subconsciously think bigger is better, so if you offer them a small cookie, they might think the small cookie was nothing special, but if you offer them a big cookie, they are so pleased to be treated lavishly. We want to be gracious hosts, so we try to make our treats grand. And we do!

People demand bigger.

We want bigger

and we're fooled into thinking that more is better.

We didn't even know that the recipe changed its serving size! We need to be mindful that portions have changed.

Some years ago, I conducted an experiment which became the documentary called *Portion Size Me*. For the experiment two graduate students were required to eat 30 days at fast restaurants, but attempt to eat the right portion for their size and physical activity level. Their food choices were tracked as were their health indicators such as liver enzyme levels during those 30 days. Because they chose the healthier options and in right portions they were able to maintain their weight – actually losing a couple of pounds, and they stayed in the healthy range for all those health markers per their doctor consults.

What the study indicated and the documentary showed was that healthy choices could be made even when eating out every meal, but the person would need to be vigilant and mindful and choose the right portion for their size and physical activity.

Section III: The Answers to the Problem

Portion Control

Everyone agrees that portions are bigger and thus are aware of the problem. But no one seems to know how to handle it. One thing my wife frequently does is put half the meal in a to-go container or apportion the meal in half before starting to eat. I look at the plate of food and I think, "I am going to save what's left." But by the time I'm done, I have eaten the whole thing.

We conducted a study to determine if this was effective by serving 18 oz. of a spaghetti dinner with a to-go box in two different conditions. The first group was given 18 oz. of spaghetti on their plate and a to-go box at the end of the meal if they wanted to take food home. They ate most of what was on their plates and saved about two ounces in their to-go box.

With the second group, we apportioned half on their plate and the other 9 oz. in the to-go box, with the instructions that if they wanted to, they could take from the box. Some people took a couple of ounces out of the to-go box to eat at the meal, but still, they saved about seven ounces.

This simple idea of taking half of our food and placing it in a to-go container before we start to eat, then spreading the remainder of the food over the plate can help us consume less when eating out when we are served large portions. The reason for this may simply be that starting with all the food on the plate, one must decide when to stop. That is very different from the second condition where a decision must be made to open the container and take more. This is more than a little bit significant. If the effort or perception of taking more is enough of a barrier to overeating, we probably need to utilize these barriers throughout the day in many settings!

Another reason for this difference in consumption may be that when we set half aside and remainder of the spaghetti is spread over the plate we feel like we have had a full portion because we start with a full plate and when we empty the plate, we've had enough. This fits the notion that a portion is whatever quantity is served, so if we are more proactive in controlling that portion, even by putting half of it aside, it will not diminish our satisfaction with the meal and provide us the sense of completion that eating all for the food on the plate does.

Affect of Pre-Meal To Go Box on Consumption

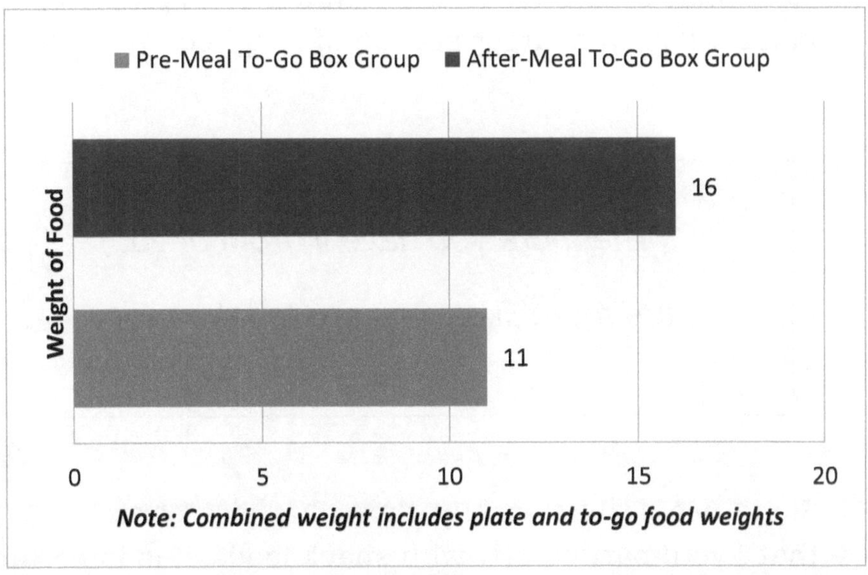

Schuster, M. J., Carlson, J. R., MacKenzie, J. A., Roche, J. D., Brooks, T. L.,Painter J. E.. (2014) Do Pre-Meal To-Go Boxes Affect the Amount of Food Consumed in a Restaurant Setting? *The Journal of the American Dietetic Association*, 113
(9 Suppl. 1), A62.

Size of Containers

Can the size of the package purchased in the grocery store effect the amount of food eaten at home, hours or even days later? Can we be unknowingly be increasing our portions at home just because of the larger size packages in the store? One study seems to say so and it didn't matter whether it was spaghetti, Crisco or

M&Ms. If we buy the larger container, when we get home, we will tend to pour or scoop more from a bigger container than if we had gotten the food from a smaller container. If we have a large container of spaghetti, our hand will grab a larger portion of spaghetti.

> *The more you have in front of you,*
>
> *the more likely you are to take **more**.*

Some people like to buy the value size container. If that's you, particularly with snack foods, it is important to apportion them after you're home into smaller packages or other small containers. It seems like a lot of trouble and yet it is an inexpensive way to make your own low calorie packages.

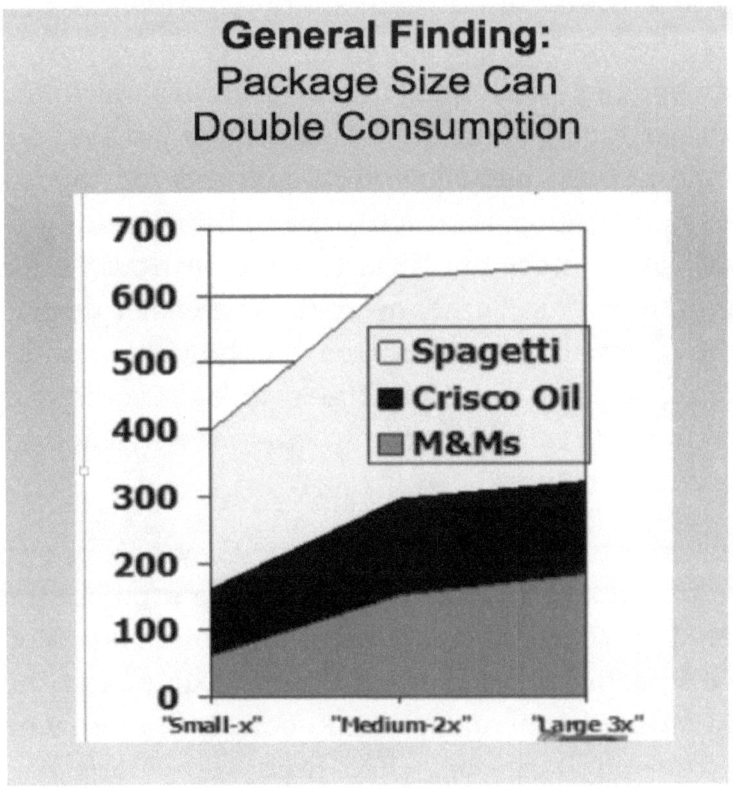

Wansink, B. (1996). Can package size accelerate usage volume? *Journal of Marketing*, 60(3), 1.

In which scenario would you eat less: eating a bag of chips with 10 portions in it, or 10 bags of chips with one portion in each?   If you keep reaching your hand into the bigger bag, you will eat substantially more. ***It is hard for us to stop eating when the large bag is open, right in front of us.*** It is easy to eat 4 portions or more in this scenario!

On the other hand, if you have a one-serving bag, and

finish it, you have to make a choice before opening up a second or a third bag. It is likely that you will eat less if you would have to get up, go to the cabinet, pull out another package and open it before eating more. Just the laziness factor alone would help us to eat less with the single portion packages. So again, having to make the decision to stop is much harder than making the decision to eat more and it is too easy in today's food environment to mindlessly overeat. The easier decision is to have small containers so we have to make a conscious decision multiple times to eat more which makes us more mindful of how much we are actually consuming.

Do 100-calorie packages work? Yes, they can but the research is mixed on how effective these are. A study published in 2011 shows that using the 100-calorie bags with people who were overweight (BMI greater than 25) and eating in the dark, would consume more when eating from one large bag than from 100-calorie bags. Interestingly, those who were in the normal BMI range (under 25) consumed about the same amount whether eating out of a larger bag or a 100-calorie bag. So is it a helpful strategy to have food items in smaller discrete portions? Yes, for people who are overweight and need to be more aware of their intake!

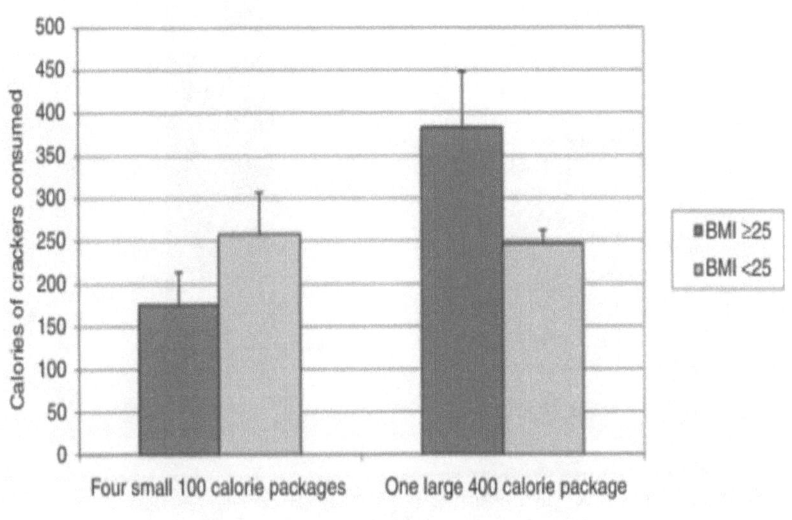

Wansink, B. , Payne, C. , & Shimizu, M. (2011). The 100-calorie semi-solution: Sub-packaging most reduces intake among the heaviest. Obesity, 19(5), 1098-1100.

The Effect of Dinnerware Size on Consumption

We have seen that the package size effects the amount of food we eat but would the same thing be true with the size of dinnerware? We've done a quite a bit of research showing cups, bowls, glasses, and spoon sizes all make a difference. It's not just at the store when we are buying something and it's not just when we are sitting in front of the TV with a bag of chips, but when we are eating at the dinner table, the size of the containers make a difference.

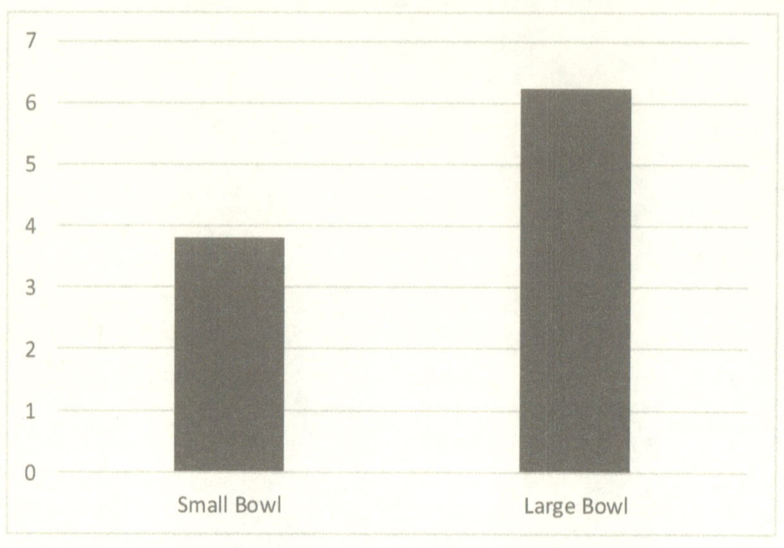

CBS Morning Show: Jim Painter & Portion-Size Me (2006)
https://www.youtube.com/watch?v=pPQdz4Gfrm8&t=128s

The ice cream study is a case in point. We gathered a convenience sample of acting students and conducted a test on the CBS Morning show regarding the effect of tableware size on consumption. People came through a self-service line and were given either a small bowl, small spoon, and small dipper, or a large bowl, spoon and dipper. In that study, the people who were provided the larger tableware ate about twice as much compared to those in the smaller tableware group. That is approximately a 50% decrease in consumption just by eating out of a smaller container with smaller utensils. They didn't miss the extra couple ozs. that the other group had.

Is there a way to know if it was all of the dinnerware that made the difference, or was one factor – the bowl, the spoon, or the dipper that made the most difference in the amount people consumed?

In doing further research, we compared 22 oz. bowls and 10 oz. bowls. We had 5ml spoons, that is, a regular teaspoon, or a   1ml tasting spoon.   We had a 4 oz. scoop and a 1 oz. scoop. We ran a similar study as above.

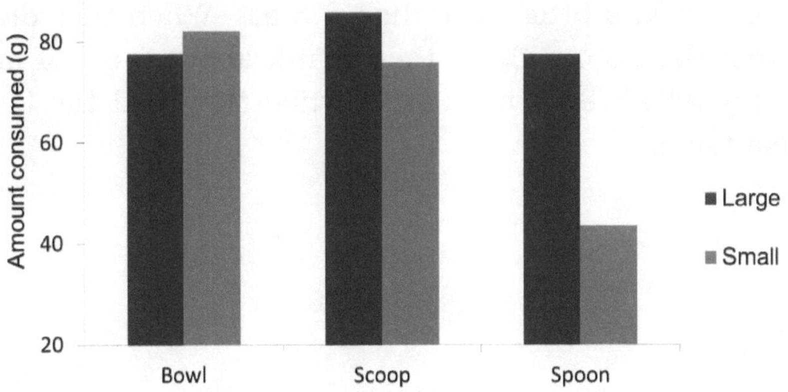

Horstmann, M. J., Merritt, J. M., Barnes, J. L., Newell, S. B., Rhodes, K., & Painter, J. E. (2011). The Effect of Dinnerware Size on Ice Cream Consumption. Journal of the American Dietetic Association, 111(9), A51-A51.

The biggest difference was not in the bowl or the scoop, but in the spoon. Was that because eating with a small spoon allowed time for satiety signals to kick in? Was it because the small spoon required more effort and time to consume the same amount?   We are not clear on that answer, but safe to say, the small spoon had an effect. If not able to implement all the changes, the utensil choice seems to be a strong factor in the effect of how much food we might eat.

But we're not always trying to eat less. Sometimes we need to eat more.   We conducted a study in 3- to 5-year-olds that varied glass size with the idea to have them to drink more milk. We gave them a 9 oz. glass or a 16 oz. glass. Now, for that age group, either glass is pretty big! When they drank from the 9 oz. glass, they consumed a little more than 3.5 oz. When they drank from the 16 oz. glass, they drank about 6 oz. of milk. They drank 80% more milk when they had the larger container.

Effect of Glass Size on Milk Consumption in Children
3 to 5 Years Old

Figure 1. Milk Consumption

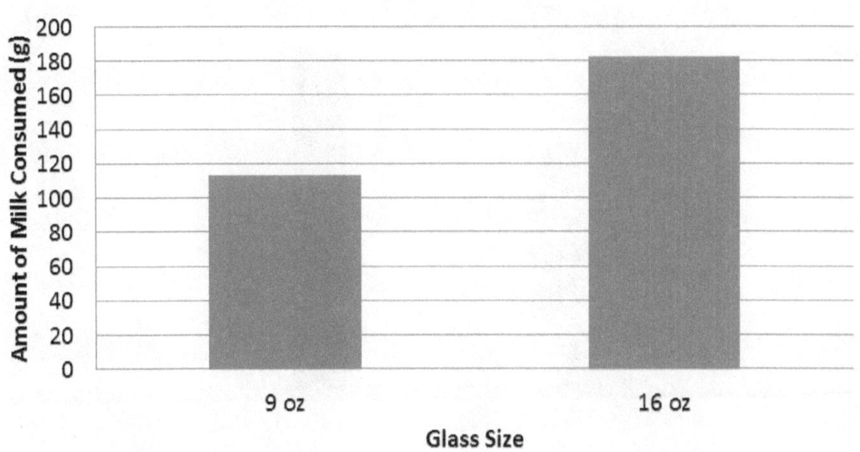

Smith, S. R., Barnes, J. L., Knoll, S. E., Rhodes, K., & Painter, J. E. (2011). Effect of Glass Size on Milk Consumption in Children 3 to 5 Years Old. Journal of the American Dietetic Association, 111(9), A106

We conducted a similar study on milk consumption with students and faculty. When the students had the larger glasses, they drank about 20% more than their smaller glass counterparts. Faculty using large glasses drank about 50% more than those using the smaller glasses.

Effect of Glass Size on Milk Consumption in Students and Faculty

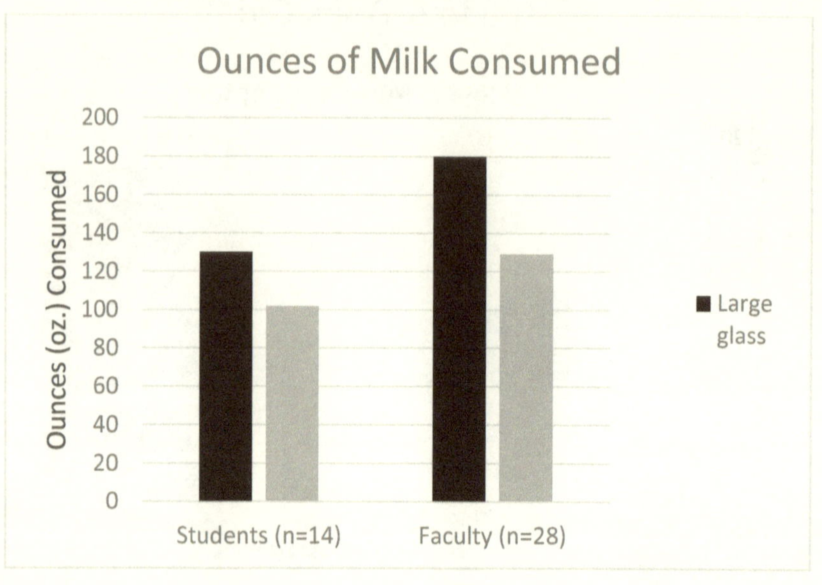

Quimby, S., O'Sullivan, C., Rhodes, K., & Painter, J. E. (2011). The Effect of Glass Size on Milk Consumption. *Journal of the American Dietetic Association,111*(9), A47-A47.

We found similar results with yogurt. If we want people to consume more yogurt, a larger container will lend them to eat more. When they had the small bowls they consumed about half as much yogurt compared to the larger bowls.

The Effect of Dinnerware Size on the Consumption of Yogurt

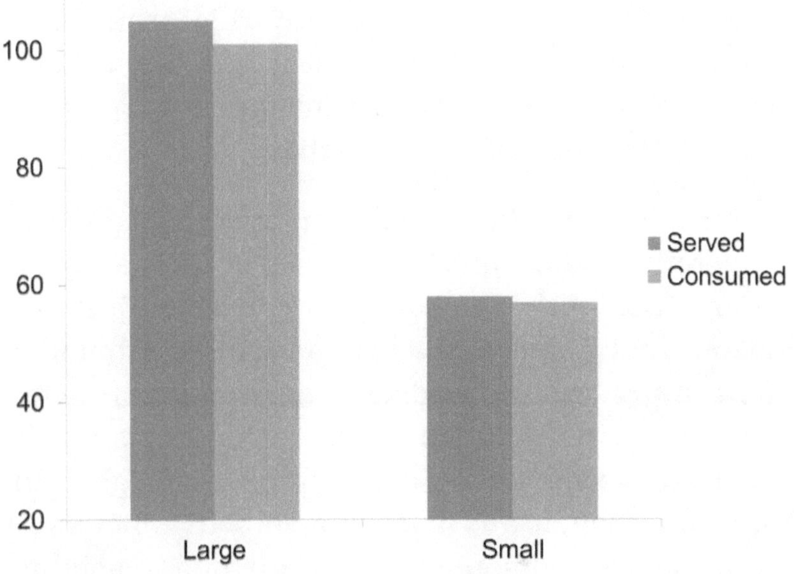

Merritt, J. M., Horstmann, M. J., Barnes, J. L., & Painter, J. E. (2011). The Effect of Dinnerware Size on the Consumption of Yogurt. Journal of the American Dietetic Association, 111(9), A91-A91.

We can apply these practices to whichever situation we are in – if we are underweight, we can choose to use bigger bowls, plates and utensils to encourage more consumption, and if we need to cut back, just changing these to a smaller size will help us achieve the goals we desire.

The Effect of Convenience on Consumption

I have always wondered, how much more candy, cookies and cakes we eat during the holiday just because they are sitting out on the counter visible and available. If something is convenient to us, and we can see it, are more likely to have more of it? This seems like an intuitive truth, but when my students did a literature search a few years ago, to my great surprise, they couldn't find any information about it.

To find out if there was an effect we conducted numerous studies. In one study we put 30 candy Kisses on an office worker's desk (very convenient), in a desk drawer, (not visible and a bit less convenient) and a few steps away from the desk (inconvenient.) On the desktop, the bowl of candy was within arm's reach. In the desk, it was just 5" below but out of sight. In the third condition, it was in a cabinet about 2 meters away, requiring the person to stand up and reach in the cabinet. When the candies were on the desk, the secretaries averaged 9 candies in a single work day. When candies were in the desk drawer, the average consumed were 6. That's amazing! It's a 30% decrease in candy consumption just by putting the candy in the drawer rather than on the desk – the difference between visible and invisible. How would you like to eat 30% less and not realize it? *The key to this is keeping it out of sight!* We tend to see food and then eat it! If we don't see it, it is out of sight and out of mind a good deal of the time. Now, just making it slightly inconvenient, to have to stand up, open a cabinet and get it decreased consumption by 60%.

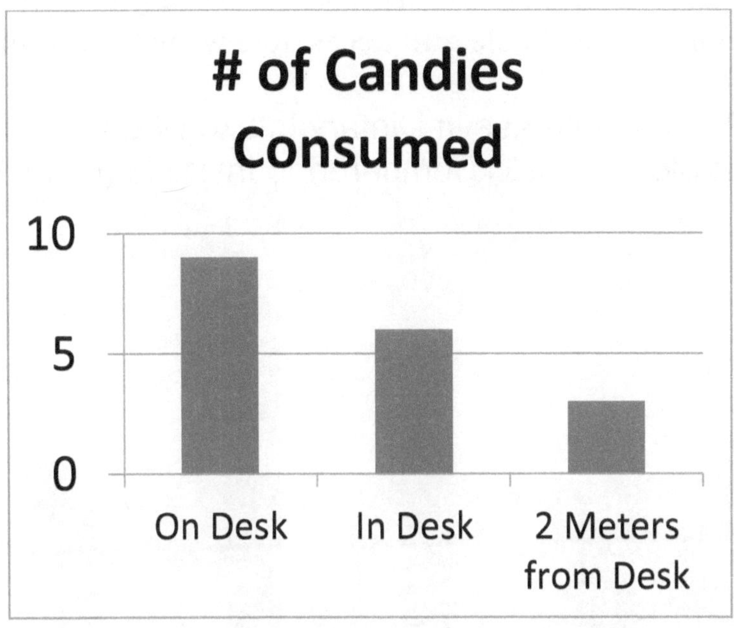

Painter, J., Wansink, B., Hieggelki, J. (2002). How Visibility and Convenience Influence Candy Consumption. Appetite 38, 237-238.

Does this principle work with healthy foods as well? We conducted a similar test with grapes, chocolates, carrots and pretzels in the desk drawer or on the desk? When we moved grapes from **in** the desk to **on** the desk, consumption increased about 15%, for chocolate and pretzels by more than 25% and carrots increased by 40%. Why did carrot consumption increase with visibility more than the others? Probably because carrots are not often a destination food that we seek out, but if they're available, we will help ourselves. We will search and seek for chocolate or pretzels, but not carrots. At 3pm, who says "I am hungry and have been craving a carrot all day." But we know they're good for us so if they're visible and accessible we will eat them.

Percent Increase in Dietary Intake when food is Visible (on desk) Compared to Invisible (in desk)

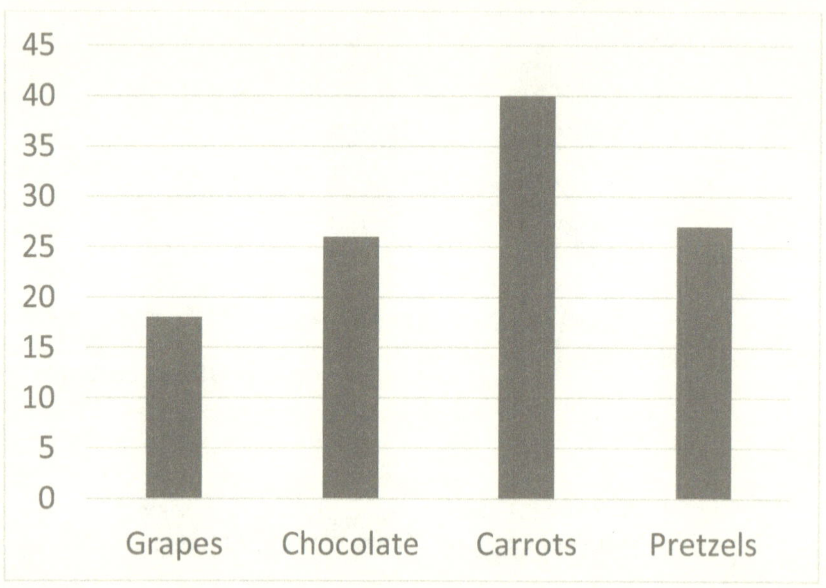

Painter, J., Snyder, J., Rhodes, K., Deisher, C. 2008. *The Effect of Visibility and Accessibility of Food on Dietary Intake*. Journal of the American Dietetic Association, 108, 9. p A93.

We conducted a similar study with raisins. We had five boxes of raisins in the desk drawer. When we moved five boxes to the desktop, consumption increased by 20%. We attempted the study again with 10 boxes instead of five and consumption increased another 20%. Visibility and ample supply added to consumption. *If we want to eat more healthy foods, make them visible and accessible.* Raisins are convenient; they don't spoil so they can sit there for a few days without a problem. When there is more of something, people eat more.

Accessibility and Visibility of Raisins

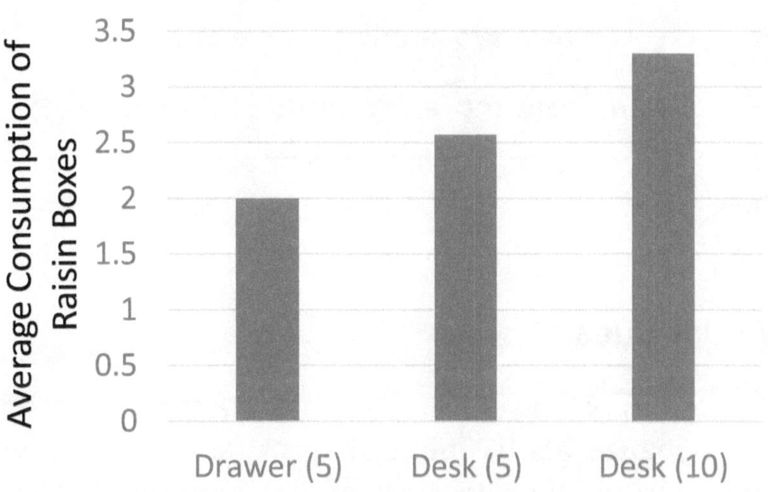

Gaydosh, B., & Painter, J. (2010). The effect of visibility and quantity of raisins on dietary intake, a pilot study. Journal of the American Dietetic Association, 110(9): A32. DOI: 10.1016/j.jada.2010.06.117.

If you have a bowl of candies in the office and there are fewer and fewer until there is one left, everyone knows it is the last one and no one wants to be the person who takes the last one. So if you pick up the last one, people seem to notice, so we tend to avoid taking the last of a thing. If there is less availability, we tend to eat less.

If there are things you want to eat less of,

make them less visible and available.

-

If there are foods you want to eat,

make them more available and accessible.

Visual Cues

This could be one of the most important aspects that we don't realize about mindfulness. Many times, visual cues tell us when to start and stop eating. If we are mindful that those cues are out there, we can use them to help us if we are not aware of them, they can hurt us.

If you buy a candy bar that is 1 or 2 oz. you'll eat the whole thing and then you're finished you are satisfied and don't eat another until the next eating occasion. You made the portion decision when you chose that size of candy. What tells you that you're done? The candy is gone! *When we see that we finished the bar, we considered that a portion and since we had that portion, we feel we have had all we need for that moment.* We usually wait an hour or a day ... some amount of time before we want another.

This effect disappears when we have the bite sized candies – the ones available around Halloween. These are small individually wrapped candies that we tend to eat en masse without a stopping place and without realizing how many we have consumed. We might have five or ten in the morning, and then another ten in the afternoon. By evening, we think we haven't eaten anything, but actually consumed 30 or more little candies. Unlike a regular sized candy that we eat one and done, we lose track of how many little candies we eat without any notion of portion.

Visual cues are very important to help us to know when to stop eating. Some years ago we did a soup study in which we had four participants at a time eating soup at a table. People could ladle out more soup if they wanted more, but none ever did. Unbeknownst to them, two of the bowls were being refilled by a tube from the pot under the table, so the level of soup didn't go down as they ate. In a normal bowl, subjects ate about 150 calories. With the refilling bowls, they ate nearly twice as much.

When asked, they thought they ate about the same amount as the others at the table showing us that we trust in visual pictures to tell us how much we've eaten. They were unaware that they had eaten so much more because the visual cue of the emptying bowl was missing!

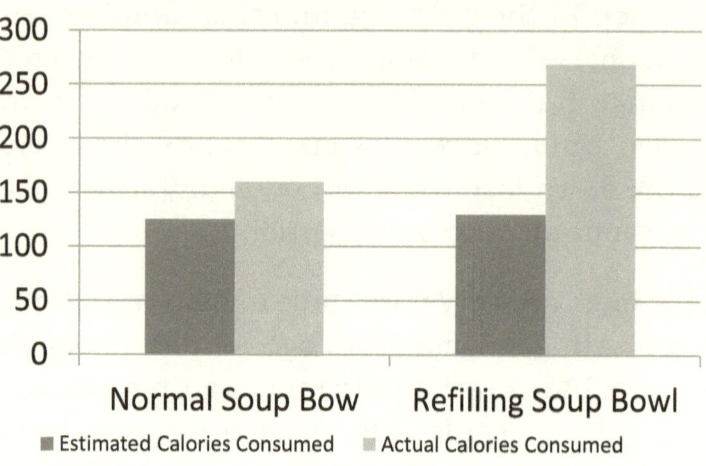

Wansink, B., Painter, JE., North, J. 2005. Bottomless Bowls: Why Visual Cues of Portion Size May Influence Intake. Obesity Research, 13,1, 93-100.

We trust that when we see a bowl, and we finish that bowl, we are done. If we lose track of that visual cue, our ability to know how much we've eaten becomes skewed. We must be mindful about visual cues that tell us how much to eat.

Can keeping empty pistachio shells visible on the desk be used as a visual cue to consumption? That is, will awareness of how much one has already consumed have any effect on whether we take more? In this study, we gave faculty members a bowl of pistachios on the desk all day and an empty bowl for the shells. The next day, we refilled the pistachios every hour and threw away the shells from the shell bowl, so the faculty lost track of how many they were eating. When the shells were visible to them, they ate about 200 calories. When the shells were cleared throughout the day, they ate about 350 calories. This is over a 50% increase when there was no evidence remaining of how much had been consumed. It's important to be mindful of the visual cues that are there.

Using Empty Pistachio Shells as Visual Cues to Consumption

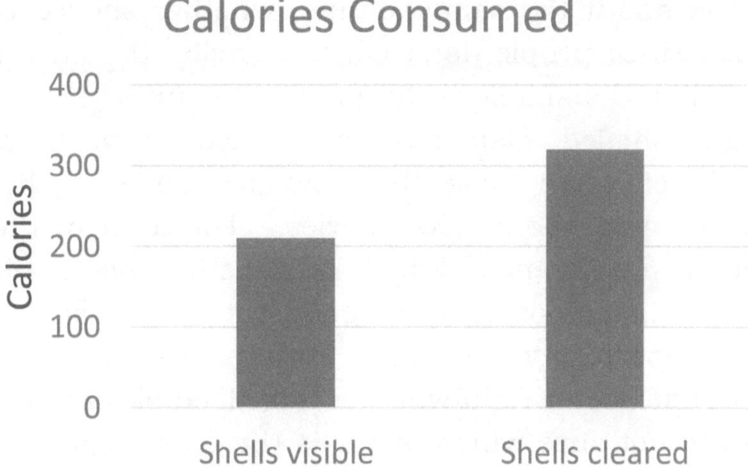

Kennedy-Hagan, K., Painter, J. E., Honselman, C., Halvorson, A., Rhodes, K., & Skwir, K. (2011). The effect of pistachio shells as a visual cue in reducing caloric consumption. Appetite, 57 (2), 418-420. doi:10.1016/j.appet.2011.06.003

The Form of the Food Influences Consumption

I have wondered if simply choosing the right form of a food would influence consumption. If a whole orange is eaten in place of orange sections will the necessity of peeling the orange cause a decrease in consumption? The same could be true for peanuts or tree nuts in the shell. To answer this question, we conducted a study with pistachios to determine if consuming nuts in the shell would reduce consumption compared to consuming shelled nuts.

As students came in to a classroom and we gave them either pistachios in the shell or shelled pistachios. They took about the same volume, whether shelled or not, but since people don't eat the shells, the ones in the shell had a smaller volume of edible nuts. Those that had shelled pistachios consumed more than 200 calories while those that had pistachios in the shell consumed about 100 calories. The form of the food made a difference. Why? Perhaps because the in-the-shell pistachios took longer to eat, satiety signals had an opportunity to kick in. Perhaps a scoop or handful portion seems right whether it is all edible or not. While I am not sure which factor is the most significant, we can determine that foods which require some kind of preparation while eating – peeling, cracking, etc., lend to lower consumption.

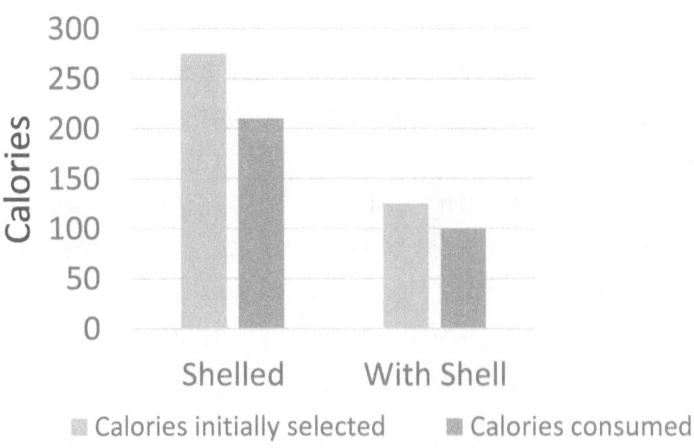

Honselman, C., Painter, J., Kennedy-Hagan, K., Halvorson, A., Rhodes, K., Brooks, T., & Skwir, K. (2011). In-shell pistachio nuts reduce caloric intake compared to shelled nuts. *Appetite, 57*(2), 414-417.

This wouldn't mean anything if the people who ate less felt hungry when they were finished so we asked if they were full or satisfied. Being unaware of whether others had consumed more or less, they told us that they were full and satisfied regardless of whether they were shelled or unshelled group. Those having to peel the shell, thus eating half of what others had consumed still **felt equally full and equally satisfied** as the ones who ate the shelled pistachios.

Words Affect Consumption

A food service director serving children K-6 once told me her story about trying to get children to eat in her cafeteria for years when she finally got an answer. The answer was to create a picture and relate the food to a pleasurable event familiar to the children. She said, "Today we are serving ball park franks; remember the ones you used to eat with dad on a warm summer evening at the baseball game and peanuts like the ones the man in the stands used to throw to you..." The children filled the lunch room.

What people are saying and what we are reading about food we eat effects our consumption. We hear the adages that talk is cheap or that words can never hurt me – basically stating that words do not have an effect. To the contrary of those adages, positive or negative messages affect us and how we feel about the foods we eat.

To see if the written word on a food label makes any difference on people's perceptions about food, we conducted a study in which people went through a cafeteria line. One day, the placard stated, "Red Beans and Rice." The next day, the placard read, "Traditional Cajun Red Beans and Rice." The first day was "Baked Fish"; the second day was "Succulent Italian Seafood Filet." We recorded what customers thought about the food offerings from one day to the next. What the customers did not know was that it was the exact same foods, prepared the same way by the same cooks. There was no difference in the actual foods.

But people reported that taste and texture were better in the ones with more descriptive names. The food tasted better when we gave names that associated it with a memory of "Grandma" or a flavor or texture like "satiny." We served "Chocolate Pudding" compared to "Grandma's Recipe Satiny Dutch Chocolate Pudding." While this also resulted in better perceptions, the labeling seemed to make a bigger difference with entrees rather than desserts, possibly because we are happy to eat a sweet dessert regardless of the description. But when it came to an entrée such as fish, taste perception improved significantly with better descriptors. On the day we served, "Baked Fish." People stated it was dry, and would catch in the throat, but when they had "Succulent Italian Seafood," they would exclaim, "I love moist, succulent fish! And who doesn't like Italian food! It's so much better than what you served before." But it was the same fish, the only thing that was different was the label.

We are more influenced

by description than we realize!

What We Say About Food Affects Our Perception of the Food

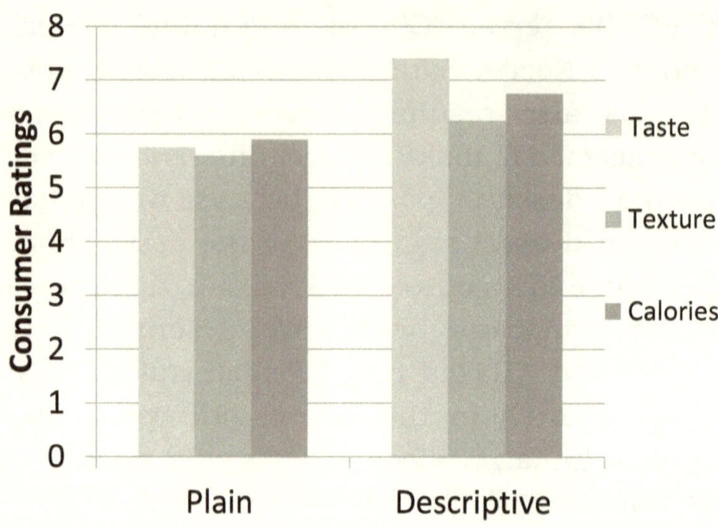

Wansink, B., Painter, J., & Ittersum, K. (2001). Descriptive menu labels' effect on sales. *The Cornell Hotel and Restaurant Administration Quarterly*, *42*(6), December 68-72.

The Effect of Descriptive Labels on Perceived Taste of Foods

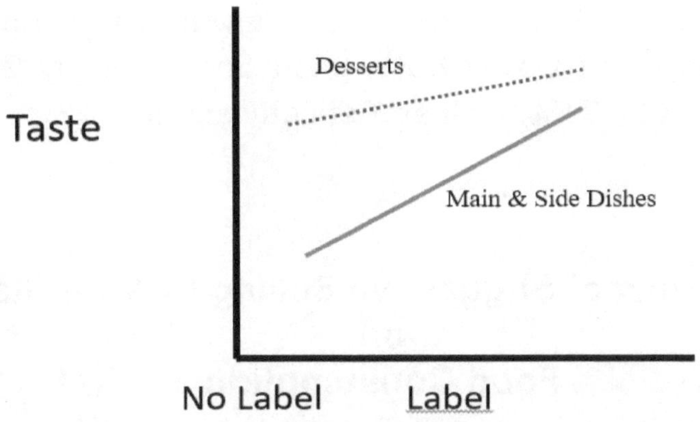

Wansink, Brian, James M. Painter, and Koert van Ittersum, (2001) "Descriptive Menu Labels' Effect on Sales," Cornell Hotel and Restaurant Administrative Quarterly, 42:6 (December), 68-72.

The above graphic depicts the increase in perceived taste when a special descriptive label was provided for the food item as differentiated from a plain label.

Suggestive Selling by Wait Staff

We also need to be especially aware when we are eating out what is said in addition to what is written about the food – what does the menu say, what does the server say? Many servers are taught to use suggestive selling.

We need to be mindful of suggestion whether it is in the printed word or spoken word. To demonstrate this, we conducted a study wherein servers were told to frequently ask one group of customers if they wanted more. A second group of consumers wasn't offered a second portion and they had to ask for one if they wanted one. When they were given suggestions, bread/rolls went up by 85%, pasta increased by 27% and cookies by 71% -- all statistically significant.

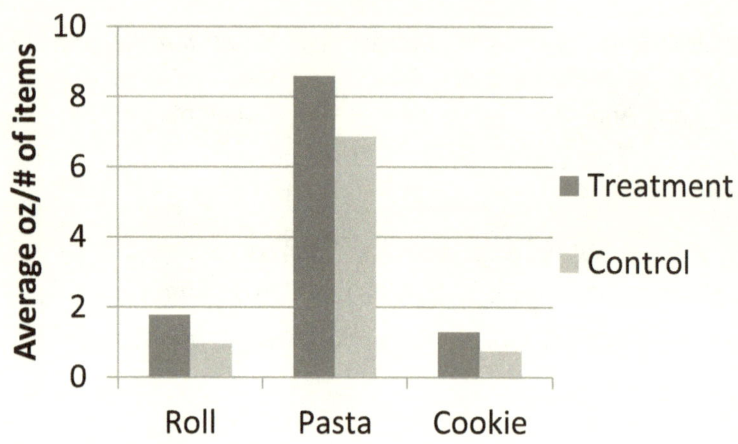

Zumwalt, G, K Kennedy-Hagan, C Honselman, K Rhodes, and J Painter. "The Effect of Suggestive Selling by Wait Staff on Food Consumption." *Journal of the American Dietetic Association*, 108.9 (2008): A39.

When we are eating at a table and have a wait staff continuing to ask if we want more, we must be mindful that suggestive selling causes us to eat more. And even worse is if they don't ask, but just keep refilling the glass of wine, for instance. It is hard to keep track of how much we are consuming when the cup never empties.   We must be mindful of suggestive selling and people pouring extra drinks.

Social Pressure

Have you ever been eating with friends at a restaurant, eyeing a special desert all night? Then when the server finally comes to take dessert orders to have your hopes dashed by a fellow diner who says "No thanks, we don't need dessert." Need… who said anything about need? No one ever needs dessert; we eat it because we want it.

I am a nutritionist who eats gluten free and thus captivated when I see flourless chocolate cake on the menu. I cannot tell you how many times my desire have been thwarted by a fellow diner when it is time for dessert by pointing to me and saying, "He is a nutritionist; we don't need dessert." Bummer, sniffle, sniffle. Why do people keep trying to associate dessert and need? This got me thinking about how much of an effect we have over the consumption of others.

We set up a study in our restaurant at the university. The study was an evening meal. Before the meal began we took one person from each table and gave them instructions to either say Yes or No the offer for second helpings. We instructed the server to ask the person we selected first at each table if they wanted seconds.

The following chart shows the consumption of the diners around the table after the first person said either Yes or No to second helpings. Look at the desserts. If the first person at the table said Yes to a second cookie, 40% of the other diners said Yes. But if the first person at the table said No to a second cookie, only 15% of the other diners at the table took seconds.

But with bread 60% of diners went for seconds whether the first person said Yes or No. Maybe there was less impact from the first diner's words for bread because there isn't the same stigma with bread as there is with dessert. It is perfectly acceptable for Americans to have more bread. Yet on the third helpings of bread the first diner saying No did seem to reduce consumption. This is in all probability not shame involved her but simply be the fatigue factor, "I'm so tired of chewing and this guy next to me doesn't want more, I don't I want any more either."

Fellow Diners Also Affect
How Much We Eat

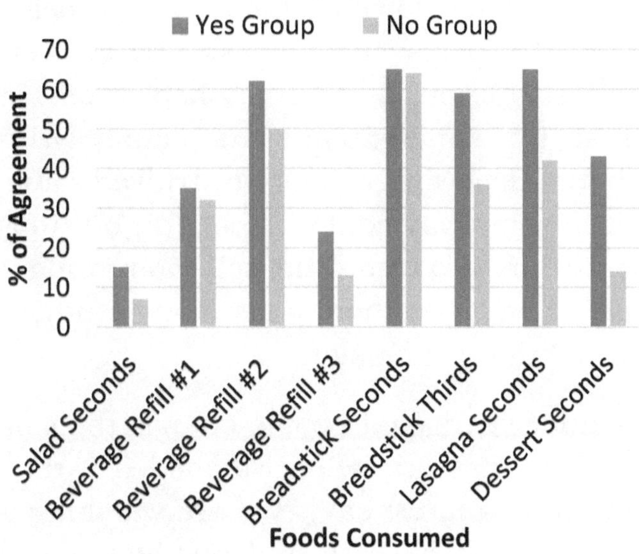

Wilcox, D., Kennedy-Hagan, K., Rhodes, K., Wilkinson, R., Painter, JE. (2008). The effect of social pressure on eating habits of college students in a restaurant environment. *Journal of the American Dietetic Association, 108 (9)*, A40.

This got me thinking. If three people ahead of us say No, No and No to dessert, is there even a possibility that we could say Yes?! I will let you know when we complete that study.

Journaling / Self-Recording

Many years ago I had an acquaintance who sat down with me at a meal. He pulled a paper out of his pocket, wrote something and put it back. I inquired about that. He said that he writes down all his food right before he eats it. He said it helps him eat less. He further told me that he lost 90 pounds and has kept it off for five years. At first, I was incredulous that simply writing it down without reviewing it for nutritive value, or analyzing it in some way could be helpful, but in going to the literature on food recording, self-monitoring really helps people to eat less, there were many studies that fully supported that conclusion.

We've known for years that people change their habits when they know they are being watched.   If they are eating something, and we say, "We are watching you," people change. It is hard to find out how and what people actually eat since they seem to want to look better for the study than they are in real life and they change the way they eat when they are being observed. If we ask them the next day to remember what they ate, selective memory comes into play. We tend to have a poor recollection of our complete intake, and especially when we try to find out a generality from the past six months. It is very difficult to find out what people are eating. But this got me thinking, although food recording doesn't give us an accurate picture of what people eat it just might be helpful to help people eat less.

There are many studies that demonstrate this. Here is a study that compares an intervention group that recorded food intake to a comparison group that didn't record. The following graph shows that the comparison group (dotted line) lost a little weight the first week of the study, but as the holidays continued they gained about two pounds until they peaked just after the holidays. The weight gain continued until a week after the holiday when either their pants didn't fit anymore or they just got tired of pigging out. This is the scenario for most of us, we gain 2 pounds during the holiday and never get it back off.

If you look at the intervention group (the solid line), in week two, they started writing down everything they ate and lost weight rapidly. The holiday began at 3.5 weeks and though they still lost some weight, it was not as much as before the holiday. Then at week 7 they stopped recording their food intake and their weight leveled off, a couple of pounds lighter than they started.

Efficacy of Self-Monitoring Food Intake

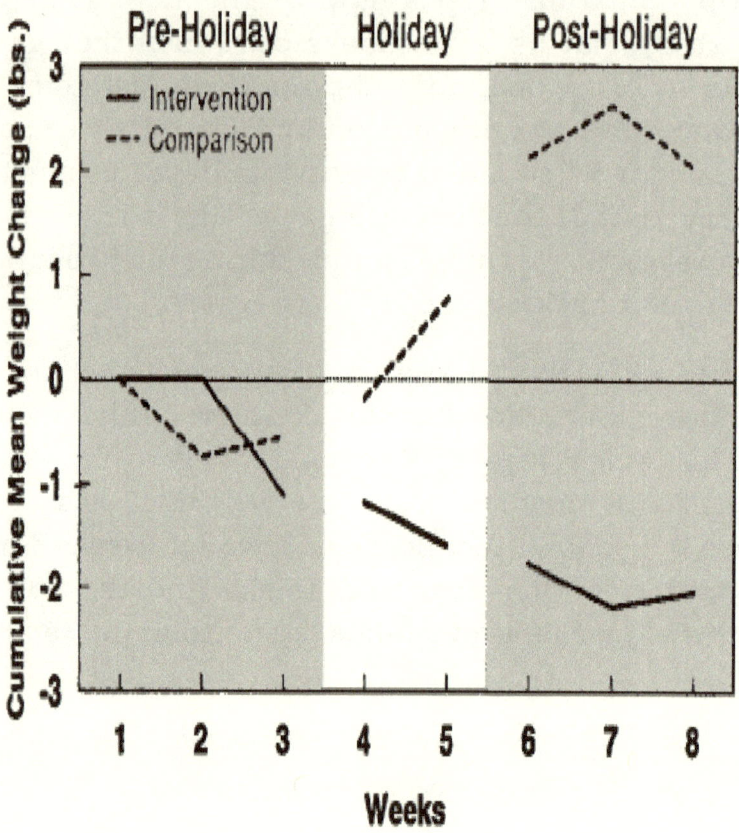

Boutelle et al. 1999, Health Psych

Self-monitoring and self-recording might be one of the most powerful mindful techniques we have available to us to help us eat less. The more you use it, the more mindful it makes you. If you write things down at the end of each week, it doesn't work. If you write it down at the end of the day, it isn't that helpful. If you write down your consumption after your meals, it is helpful, but it is most helpful to write it down **just before** you eat – right before you put it in your mouth!

You pull out your paper; have it in front of you, write it down and then eat because then you **have a chance to look and possibly change** what you might be getting ready to eat. For instance, you might see a list of what you've already eaten and say to yourself, "Oh Wow! Look at that list! I've had a lot already!" and then have less in the next moment on purpose.

Giving yourself a chance at the point of consumption to say No, Not Now – is a great technique. It doesn't deny you forever. You can eat it in a few minutes or hours or days, but the point is the ability to pass up extra calories one moment at a time.

Conclusion

When we approach eating with a sense of mindfulness beyond the immediate sensory perceptions, we may be able to change the amounts of food that we consume. As we become more mindful about situations and messages that influence our consumption, we may be able to reduce eating out of boredom or stress, not mindlessly gobbling up everything in front of us. Here's to healthier us!

This text is not a systematic review of the subject of mindful eating, or even a definitive study of the subject. It is not intended to be scientific proof of the matter. What it does provide is a list of mindful eating tips that are research-based.

Practical Tips

Be mindful when

Shopping: Smaller packages may decrease consumption and portion pack items are even more helpful.

Snacking: If we put our hands into smaller containers we may eat less.

Eating at home: Swap out the larger plates, bowls, glasses and even flatware for smaller ones will encourage consumption to decrease. Keep foods that are temptations out of sight and healthier foods you want to consume in sight. Keeping food at a distance and less accessible may decrease consumption.

Eating out: put half of the meal in a to-go box before you start eating. Spread the rest of the meal over the plate and enjoy. You help yourself and influence others to eat less by turning down second portions before anyone else speaks. Be aware that what people say and what is written about food will affect your perception and may encourage overeating.

At all times: Be aware of visual cues to consumption, record what you eat and review before each eating occasion.

References

Baker and Kirschenbaum, 1998, Health Psych

Boutelle et al. 1999, Health Psych

Edwards, A. (2012, June 06). At 7-Eleven, the Big Gulps Elude a Ban by the City. Retrieved December 28, 2016. <u>Web</u>

Gaydosh, B., & Painter, J. (2010). The effect of visibility and quantity of raisins on dietary intake, a pilot study. *Journal of the American Dietetic Association*, 110(9): A32. DOI: 10.1016/j.jada.2010.06.117.

Honselman, C., Painter, J., Kennedy-Hagan, K., Halvorson, A., Rhodes, K., Brooks, T., & Skwir, K. (2011). In-shell pistachio nuts reduce caloric intake compared to shelled nuts. *Appetite*, 57(2), 414-417

Horstmann, M. J., Merritt, J. M., Barnes, J. L., Newell, S. B., Rhodes, K., & Painter, J. E. (2011). The Effect of Dinnerware Size on Ice Cream Consumption. *Journal of the American Dietetic Association*, 111(9), A51-A51.

Kennedy-Hagan, K., Painter, J. E., Honselman, C.,Halvorson, A., Rhodes, K., & Skwir, K. (2011). The effect of pistachio shells as a visual cue in reducing caloric consumption. *Appetite*, 57 (2), 418-420. doi:10.1016/j.appet.2011.06.003

McDonald's Nutrition Calculator | McDonald's. (n.d.). Retrieved from <u>Web</u>

Merritt, J. M., Horstmann, M. J., Barnes, J. L., & Painter, J. E. (2011). The Effect of Dinnerware Size on the Consumption of Yogurt. *Journal of the American Dietetic Association*, 111(9), A91-A91.

Monster Burger Calories, NBC News (2004). Retrieved from <u>Web</u>

Norton, A. (2016, December 13). Fewer Babies in Poor Families Are Overweight: CDC. Retrieved from <u>Web</u>

Painter, J., Snyder, J., Rhodes, K., Deisher, C. 2008. The Effect of Visibility and Accessibility of Food on Dietary Intake. *Journal of the American Dietetic Association*, 108, 9. p A93.

Painter, J., Wansink, B., Hieggelki, J. (2002). How Visibility and Convenience Influence Candy Consumption. *Appetite* 38, 237-238.

Portion Distribution I. (2003). Retrieved from <u>Web</u>

Portion Distribution II. (2004). Retrieved from <u>Web</u>

Quality Is Our Recipe. (n.d.). Retrieved from <u>Web</u>

Quimby, S., O'Sullivan, C., Rhodes, K., & Painter, J. E. (2011). The Effect of Glass Size on Milk Consumption. *Journal of the American Dietetic Association*,111(9), A47-A47.

Schuster, M. J., Carlson, J. R., MacKenzie, J. A., Roche, J. D., Brooks, T. L., Painter J. E.. (2014) Do Pre-Meal To-Go Boxes Affect the Amount of Food Consumed in a Restaurant Setting? *The Journal of the American Dietetic Association*, 113(9 Suppl. 1), A62.

Smith, S. R., Barnes, J. L., Knoll, S. E., Rhodes, K., & Painter, J. E. (2011). Effect of Glass Size on Milk Consumption in Children 3 to 5 Years Old. *Journal of the American Dietetic Association*, 111(9), A106-A106.

The **Wall** Street Journal. 2013. Judge Cans Soda Ban. Retrieved from <u>Web</u>

Wansink, B. (1996). Can package size accelerate usage volume?. *Journal of Marketing*, *60*(3), 1.

Wansink, B. , Painter, J. , & Ittersum, K. (2001). Descriptive menu labels' effect on sales. *The Cornell Hotel and Restaurant Administration Quarterly*, *42*(6), December 68-72.

Wansink, B. , Payne, C. , & Shimizu, M. (2011). The 100-calorie semi-solution: Sub-packaging most reduces intake among the heaviest. *Obesity*, 19(5), 1098-1100.

Wansink, B., Painter, J.E., North, J. 2005. Bottomless Bowls: Why Visual Cues of Portion Size May Influence Intake. *Obesity Research*, 13,1, 93-100.

WHO | World Health Organization. (n.d.). Retrieved from <u>Web</u>

Wilcox, D. , Kennedy-Hagan, K. , Rhodes, K. , Wilkinson, R. , & Painter, J. (2008). The effect of social pressure on the eating habits of college students in a restaurant environment. *Journal of the American Dietetic Association*, 108(9), A40.

Young & Nestle, 2003. JADA Expanding Portion Sizes in the US Marketplace. (231-234)

Zumwalt, G., Kennedy-Hagan, K., Honselman, C., Rhodes, K., and J Painter. "The Effect of Suggestive Selling by Wait Staff on Food Consumption." *Journal of the American Dietetic Association*, 108.9 (2008): A39